**This Logbook Belongs To:**

---

City – State – Country:

---

Phone Number and Email:

---

Physician and Contact Information:

---

Emergency Contact Person and Phone Number:

---



Reviewed by Dr. D.I. Doughan, University Professor

 ISBN: 978-1-952966-10-1

CONTACTtracingLOG@gmail.com

## WHAT IS CONTACT TRACING?

Contact tracing is a public health strategy used to interrupt the spreading of an infectious disease. It begins with talking to the "person of interest" and finding out who they had physical contact with in the past several weeks. It then traces those contacts, has them tested for the infection, and treats them. This process is then repeated with each contact exposed to the infection. Contact tracing supports the public health goal of reducing infections in a community.

The goals of contact tracing are:

- To interrupt the transmission patterns thus reducing the spread of an infection in the community;
- To alert "persons of interest" to the possibility of infection and then offer proactive and preventive counseling;
- To offer diagnosis, counseling, and treatment to infected individuals;
- To prevent the person from being infected again if possible;
- To learn more about how a disease impacts a specific community and this knowledge helps to manage and contain how a disease spreads.

Contact tracing is a critical step for disease control in public health. It manages the spread of a disease by addressing community transmission.

Historically, disease epidemics and pandemics – such as Smallpox, Tuberculosis, Ebola, HIV, Measles, and SARS – were largely managed by using exhaustive contact tracing efforts that located all infected individuals and their contacts.

For contact tracing to be effective, the majority of a community needs to participate in the effort.

## ABOUT THE AUTHORS & LOG

This logbook was written by Dr. J.A. Talkington who earned a PhD in Environmental Science at Oklahoma State University in the USA. Dr. Talkington has also studied disease symptomatology, toxicology, graphic design, and historical research methods. Dr. Talkington is known as a science historian, a business professor, a health researcher, and a certified contact tracer.

This logbook was co-authored by Dr. N. S. Najd who earned a PhD in Industrial Engineering and Management at Oklahoma State University in the USA. Dr. Najd has also studied civil and environmental engineering, systems thinking, English, Arabic, and French. Dr. Najd is known as a project manager, a quality consultant, an interdisciplinary and sustainability professor, a higher education administrator, and a certified contact tracer.

This logbook was conceived by Dr. Talkington after an email exchange discussing contact tracing with a researcher at the Centers for Disease Control (CDC). It is vital for the 'person of interest' to be able to identify who they have been in contact with during the previous several weeks. This likely requires maintaining a written record of their interactions with people. If the 'person of interest' cannot recall *all* of their interactions, critical information will be lost and the public will be endangered further.

Given the privacy concerns about using cellular telephone data to monitor users' movements, a paperback logbook seemed a logical and necessary solution.Recognizing the need, Dr. Talkington created the *Contact Tracing Log – A Logical Necessity*™.
This book of forms allows a person to log vital information about their travels and their interactions with other people. The *Contact Tracing Log – A Logical Necessity*™ is available as a paperback book in various sizes and multiple languages on Amazon websites worldwide.



ISBN: 978-1-952966-10-1

CONTACTtracingLOG@gmail.com

**your health:**
Slight headache at
8 am, Super now

| PLACE & address | NAMES include people you traveled with | mask on others yes no | Arrival time | Departure time | washed hands before yes no | hand sanitizer before yes no | mask on you yes no | transportation | body temperature | outdoors or inside | # of people | washed hands after yes no | hand sanitizer after yes no |
|---|---|---|---|---|---|---|---|---|---|---|---|---|---|
| Eskimo Joe's™ Elm & Duck | Bob V. | N | 10:30 AM | 12:15 PM | Y | N | Y | Car | 98.6 | i | 12 | N | Y |
| | Donald | N | | | | | | | | | | | |
| | Trish, server | Y | | | | | | | | | | | |
| post Office 8th & Lewis | Mr. Townsend | Y | 12:15 PM | 12:30 PM | N | Y | Y | WALK | | i | 7 | N | Y |

describe the social distancing





**DATE:** TUES - July 7, 2020

hand sanitizer after yes no

washed hands after yes no

# of people

outdoors or inside

body temperature

transportation

DATE:

mask on you yes no

hand sanitizer before yes no

washed hands before yes no

Departure time

Arrival time

mask on others yes no

your health:

NAMES include people you traveled with

describe the social distancing

PLACE & address

hand sanitizer after yes no

washed hands after yes no

# of people

outdoors or inside

body temperature

transportation

mask on you yes no

hand sanitizer before yes no

washed hands before yes no

Departure time

Arrival time

mask on others yes no

your health:

PLACE
& address

NAMES
include people you traveled with

describe the social distancing

DATE:

hand sanitizer after yes no

washed hands after yes no

# of people

outdoors or inside

body temperature

transportation

mask on you yes no

hand sanitizer before yes no

washed hands before yes no

**Departure time**

**Arrival time**

mask on others yes no

**DATE:**

**your health:**

**PLACE**
& address

**NAMES**
include people you traveled with

**describe the social distancing**

hand sanitizer after yes no

washed hands after yes no

# of people

outdoors or inside

body temperature

transportation

mask on you yes no

hand sanitizer before yes no

washed hands before yes no

**Departure time**

**Arrival time**

mask on others yes no

**your health:**

**NAMES** include people you traveled with

**PLACE** & address

**describe the social distancing**

**DATE:**

hand sanitizer after yes no

washed hands after yes no

# of people

outdoors or inside

body temperature

transportation

mask on you yes no

hand sanitizer before yes no

washed hands before yes no

Departure time

Arrival time

mask on others yes no

**DATE:**

describe the social distancing

**NAMES**
include people you traveled with

**PLACE**
& address

your health:

DATE:

**PLACE** & address

**NAMES** include people you traveled with

**your health:**

describe the social distancing

mask on others yes no

**Arrival time**

**Departure time**

washed hands before yes no

hand sanitizer before yes no

mask on you yes no

transportation

body temperature

outdoors or inside

# of people

washed hands after yes no

hand sanitizer after yes no

your health:

**PLACE**
& address

**NAMES**
include people you traveled with

describe the social distancing

mask on others yes no

**Arrival time**

**Departure time**

washed hands before yes no

hand sanitizer before yes no

mask on you yes no

transportation

body temperature

outdoors or inside

# of people

washed hands after yes no

hand sanitizer after yes no

**DATE:**

your health:

**PLACE**
& address

**NAMES**
include people
you traveled with

describe the
social distancing

mask on others yes no

**Arrival time**

**Departure time**

washed hands before yes no

hand sanitizer before yes no

mask on you yes no

transportation

body temperature

outdoors or inside

# of people

washed hands after yes no

hand sanitizer after yes no

**DATE:**

hand sanitizer after yes no

washed hands after yes no

# of people

outdoors or inside

body temperature

transportation

DATE:

mask on you yes no

hand sanitizer before yes no

washed hands before yes no

Departure time

Arrival time

mask on others yes no

your health:

NAMES
include people you traveled with

describe the social distancing

PLACE
& address

hand sanitizer after yes no

washed hands after yes no

# of people

outdoors or inside

body temperature

transportation

mask on you yes no

hand sanitizer before yes no

washed hands before yes no

**Departure time**

**Arrival time**

mask on others yes no

your health:

**NAMES**
include people you traveled with

**PLACE**
& address

describe the social distancing

**DATE:**

hand sanitizer after yes no

washed hands after yes no

# of people

outdoors or inside

body temperature

transportation

mask on you yes no

hand sanitizer before yes no

washed hands before yes no

Departure time

Arrival time

mask on others yes no

DATE:

your health:

NAMES
include people you traveled with

PLACE
& address

describe the social distancing

your health:

| PLACE & address | NAMES include people you traveled with | mask on others yes no | Arrival time | Departure time | washed hands before yes no | hand sanitizer before yes no | mask on you yes no | transportation | body temperature | outdoors or inside | # of people | washed hands after yes no | hand sanitizer after yes no |
|---|---|---|---|---|---|---|---|---|---|---|---|---|---|
| | | | | | | | | | | | | | |

describe the social distancing



DATE:

DATE:

hand sanitizer after yes no

washed hands after yes no

# of people

outdoors or inside

body temperature

transportation

mask on you yes no

hand sanitizer before yes no

washed hands before yes no

**Departure time**

**Arrival time**

mask on others yes no

describe the social distancing

your health:

**NAMES** include people you traveled with

**PLACE** & address

hand sanitizer after yes no

washed hands after yes no

# of people

outdoors or inside

body temperature

transportation

mask on you yes no

hand sanitizer before yes no

washed hands before yes no

Departure time

Arrival time

mask on others yes no

DATE:

**PLACE** & address

**NAMES** include people you traveled with

your health:

describe the social distancing

your health:

PLACE & address

NAMES include people you traveled with

mask on others yes no

Arrival time

Departure time

washed hands before yes no

hand sanitizer before yes no

mask on you yes no

transportation

body temperature

outdoors or inside

# of people

washed hands after yes no

hand sanitizer after yes no

DATE:

describe the social distancing

hand sanitizer after yes no

washed hands after yes no

# of people

outdoors or inside

body temperature

transportation

mask on you yes no

hand sanitizer before yes no

washed hands before yes no

Departure time

Arrival time

mask on others yes no

your health:

**PLACE**
& address

**NAMES**
include people you traveled with

describe the social distancing

DATE:

hand sanitizer after yes no

washed hands after yes no

# of people

outdoors or inside

body temperature

transportation

mask on you yes no

hand sanitizer before yes no

washed hands before yes no

**Departure time**

**Arrival time**

mask on others yes no

DATE:

your health:

**NAMES**
include people you traveled with

**PLACE**
& address

describe the social distancing

hand sanitizer after yes no

washed hands after yes no

# of people

outdoors or inside

body temperature

transportation

mask on you yes no

hand sanitizer before yes no

washed hands before yes no

Departure time

Arrival time

mask on others yes no

DATE:

your health:

PLACE & address

NAMES include people you traveled with

describe the social distancing

DATE:

hand sanitizer after yes no

washed hands after yes no

# of people

outdoors or inside

body temperature

transportation

mask on you yes no

hand sanitizer before yes no

washed hands before yes no

**Departure time**

**Arrival time**

mask on others yes no

describe the social distancing

**NAMES** include people you traveled with

**PLACE** & address

your health:

hand sanitizer after yes no

washed hands after yes no

\# of people

outdoors or inside

body temperature

transportation

mask on you yes no

hand sanitizer before yes no

washed hands before yes no

**Departure time**

**Arrival time**

mask on others yes no

**your health:**

**PLACE** & address

**NAMES** include people you traveled with

**describe the social distancing**

**DATE:**

hand sanitizer after yes no

washed hands after yes no

# of people

outdoors or inside

body temperature

transportation

mask on you yes no

hand sanitizer before yes no

washed hands before yes no

Departure time

Arrival time

mask on others yes no

your health:

NAMES
include people you traveled with

describe the social distancing

PLACE
& address

DATE:

hand sanitizer after yes no

washed hands after yes no

# of people

outdoors or inside

body temperature

transportation

mask on you yes no

hand sanitizer before yes no

washed hands before yes no

**Departure time**

**Arrival time**

mask on others yes no

your health:

**NAMES** include people you traveled with

**PLACE** & address

describe the social distancing

DATE:

your health:

| PLACE & address | NAMES include people you traveled with | mask on others yes no | Arrival time | Departure time | washed hands before yes no | hand sanitizer before yes no | mask on you yes no | transportation | body temperature | outdoors or inside | # of people | washed hands after yes no | hand sanitizer after yes no |
|---|---|---|---|---|---|---|---|---|---|---|---|---|---|
| | describe the social distancing | | | | | | | | | | | | |



DATE:

hand sanitizer after yes no

washed hands after yes no

# of people

outdoors or inside

body temperature

transportation

mask on you yes no

hand sanitizer before yes no

washed hands before yes no

**Departure time**

**Arrival time**

mask on others yes no

**your health:**

**PLACE** & address

**NAMES** include people you traveled with

**describe the social distancing**

**DATE:**

DATE:

hand sanitizer after yes no

washed hands after yes no

# of people

outdoors or inside

body temperature

transportation

mask on you yes no

hand sanitizer before yes no

washed hands before yes no

**Departure time**

**Arrival time**

mask on others yes no

your health:

**NAMES**
include people
you traveled with

**PLACE**
& address

describe the
social distancing

your health:

| PLACE & address | NAMES include people you traveled with | mask on others yes no | Arrival time | Departure time | washed hands before yes no | hand sanitizer before yes no | mask on you yes no | transportation | body temperature | outdoors or inside | # of people | washed hands after yes no | hand sanitizer after yes no |
|---|---|---|---|---|---|---|---|---|---|---|---|---|---|
| | describe the social distancing | | | | | | | | | | | | |



DATE:

DATE:

PLACE & address

NAMES include people you traveled with

mask on others yes no

Arrival time

Departure time

washed hands before yes no

hand sanitizer before yes no

mask on you yes no

transportation

body temperature

outdoors or inside

# of people

washed hands after yes no

hand sanitizer after yes no

describe the social distancing

your health:

DATE:

your health:

PLACE
& address

NAMES
include people
you traveled with

describe the
social distancing

| | |
|---|---|
| hand sanitizer after | yes no |
| washed hands after | yes no |
| # of people | |
| outdoors or inside | |
| body temperature | |
| transportation | |
| mask on you | yes no |
| hand sanitizer before | yes no |
| washed hands before | yes no |
| Departure time | |
| Arrival time | |
| mask on others | yes no |

hand sanitizer after yes no

washed hands after yes no

# of people

outdoors or inside

body temperature

transportation

mask on you yes no

hand sanitizer before yes no

washed hands before yes no

**Departure time**

**Arrival time**

mask on others yes no

**DATE:**

your health:

**NAMES**
include people you traveled with

**PLACE**
& address

describe the social distancing

DATE:

| PLACE & address | NAMES include people you traveled with | mask on others yes no | Arrival time | Departure time | washed hands before yes no | hand sanitizer before yes no | mask on you yes no | transportation | body temperature | outdoors or inside | # of people | washed hands after yes no | hand sanitizer after yes no |
|---|---|---|---|---|---|---|---|---|---|---|---|---|---|
| | | | | | | | | | | | | | |

your health:

describe the social distancing

hand sanitizer after yes no

washed hands after yes no

# of people

outdoors or inside

body temperature

transportation

mask on you yes no

hand sanitizer before yes no

washed hands before yes no

**Departure time**

**Arrival time**

mask on others yes no

**NAMES**
include people you traveled with

**PLACE**
& address

your health:

describe the social distancing

**DATE:**

your health:

| PLACE & address | NAMES include people you traveled with | mask on others yes no | Arrival time | Departure time | washed hands before yes no | hand sanitizer before yes no | mask on you yes no | transportation | body temperature | outdoors or inside | # of people | washed hands after yes no | hand sanitizer after yes no |
|---|---|---|---|---|---|---|---|---|---|---|---|---|---|
| | describe the social distancing | | | | | | | | | | | | |



DATE:

hand sanitizer after yes no

washed hands after yes no

# of people

outdoors or inside

body temperature

transportation

mask on you yes no

hand sanitizer before yes no

washed hands before yes no

Departure time

Arrival time

mask on others yes no

your health:

PLACE
& address

NAMES
include people you traveled with

describe the social distancing

DATE:

DATE:

hand sanitizer after yes no

washed hands after yes no

# of people

outdoors or inside

body temperature

transportation

mask on you yes no

hand sanitizer before yes no

washed hands before yes no

Departure time

Arrival time

mask on others yes no

your health:

PLACE & address

NAMES include people you traveled with

describe the social distancing

DATE:

**PLACE**
& address

**NAMES**
include people you traveled with

mask on others yes no

**Arrival time**

**Departure time**

washed hands before yes no

hand sanitizer before yes no

mask on you yes no

transportation

body temperature

outdoors or inside

# of people

washed hands after yes no

hand sanitizer after yes no

your health:

describe the social distancing

DATE:

hand sanitizer after yes no

washed hands after yes no

# of people

outdoors or inside

body temperature

transportation

mask on you yes no

hand sanitizer before yes no

washed hands before yes no

Departure time

Arrival time

mask on others yes no

your health:

PLACE & address

NAMES include people you traveled with

describe the social distancing

DATE:

hand sanitizer after yes no

washed hands after yes no

# of people

outdoors or inside

body temperature

transportation

mask on you yes no

hand sanitizer before yes no

washed hands before yes no

## Departure time

## Arrival time

mask on others yes no

describe the social distancing

your health:

**NAMES** include people you traveled with

**PLACE** & address

**DATE:**

**your health:**

**PLACE** & address

**NAMES** include people you traveled with

mask on others yes no

**Arrival time**

**Departure time**

washed hands before yes no

hand sanitizer before yes no

mask on you yes no

transportation

body temperature

outdoors or inside

# of people

washed hands after yes no

hand sanitizer after yes no

describe the social distancing

hand sanitizer after yes no

washed hands after yes no

# of people

outdoors or inside

body temperature

transportation

mask on you yes no

hand sanitizer before yes no

washed hands before yes no

Departure time

Arrival time

mask on others yes no

your health:

NAMES
include people you traveled with

PLACE
& address

describe the social distancing

DATE:

your health:

| PLACE & address | NAMES include people you traveled with | mask on others yes no | Arrival time | Departure time | washed hands before yes no | hand sanitizer before yes no | mask on you yes no | transportation | body temperature | outdoors or inside | # of people | washed hands after yes no | hand sanitizer after yes no |
|---|---|---|---|---|---|---|---|---|---|---|---|---|---|
| | describe the social distancing | | | | | | | | | | | | |



DATE:

hand sanitizer after yes no

washed hands after yes no

\# of people

outdoors or inside

body temperature

transportation

mask on you yes no

hand sanitizer before yes no

washed hands before yes no

Departure time

Arrival time

mask on others yes no

your health:

NAMES
include people you traveled with

PLACE
& address

describe the social distancing

DATE:

hand sanitizer after yes no

washed hands after yes no

# of people

outdoors or inside

body temperature

transportation

mask on you yes no

hand sanitizer before yes no

washed hands before yes no

Departure time

Arrival time

mask on others yes no

DATE:

your health:

PLACE
& address

NAMES
include people you traveled with

describe the social distancing

DATE:

your health:

PLACE
& address

NAMES
include people
you traveled with

describe the
social distancing

mask on others yes no

Arrival time

Departure time

washed hands before yes no

hand sanitizer before yes no

mask on you yes no

transportation

body temperature

outdoors or inside

# of people

washed hands after yes no

hand sanitizer after yes no

DATE:

**PLACE** & address

**NAMES** include people you traveled with

**mask on others** yes no

**Arrival time**

**Departure time**

**washed hands before** yes no

**hand sanitizer before** yes no

**mask on you** yes no

**transportation**

**body temperature**

**outdoors or inside**

**# of people**

**washed hands after** yes no

**hand sanitizer after** yes no

**describe the social distancing**

**your health:**

hand sanitizer after yes no

washed hands after yes no

# of people

outdoors or inside

body temperature

transportation

mask on you yes no

hand sanitizer before yes no

washed hands before yes no

Departure time

Arrival time

mask on others yes no

your health:

NAMES
include people you traveled with

PLACE
& address

describe the social distancing

DATE:

hand sanitizer after yes no

washed hands after yes no

# of people

outdoors or inside

body temperature

transportation

mask on you yes no

hand sanitizer before yes no

washed hands before yes no

**Departure time**

**Arrival time**

mask on others yes no

DATE:

your health:

**PLACE**
& address

**NAMES**
include people you traveled with

describe the social distancing

DATE:

your health:

**PLACE**
& address

**NAMES**
include people
you traveled with

describe the
social distancing

mask on others yes no

**Arrival time**

**Departure time**

washed hands before yes no

hand sanitizer before yes no

mask on you yes no

transportation

body temperature

outdoors or inside

# of people

washed hands after yes no

hand sanitizer after yes no

DATE:

hand sanitizer after yes no

washed hands after yes no

# of people

outdoors or inside

body temperature

transportation

mask on you yes no

hand sanitizer before yes no

washed hands before yes no

Departure time

Arrival time

mask on others yes no

your health:

PLACE & address

NAMES include people you traveled with

describe the social distancing

hand sanitizer after yes no

washed hands after yes no

# of people

outdoors or inside

body temperature

transportation

mask on you yes no

hand sanitizer before yes no

washed hands before yes no

Departure time

Arrival time

mask on others yes no

DATE:

your health:

NAMES
include people you traveled with

PLACE
& address

describe the social distancing

DATE:

PLACE & address

NAMES include people you traveled with

your health:

describe the social distancing

mask on others yes no

Arrival time

Departure time

washed hands before yes no

hand sanitizer before yes no

mask on you yes no

transportation

body temperature

outdoors or inside

# of people

washed hands after yes no

hand sanitizer after yes no

hand sanitizer after yes no

washed hands after yes no

# of people

outdoors or inside

body temperature

transportation

mask on you yes no

hand sanitizer before yes no

washed hands before yes no

**Departure time**

**Arrival time**

mask on others yes no

your health:

**NAMES**
include people you traveled with

**PLACE**
& address

describe the social distancing

DATE:

hand sanitizer after yes no

washed hands after yes no

# of people

outdoors or inside

body temperature

transportation

mask on you yes no

hand sanitizer before yes no

washed hands before yes no

**Departure time**

**Arrival time**

mask on others yes no

**your health:**

**PLACE**
& address

**NAMES**
include people you traveled with

describe the social distancing

**DATE:**

DATE:

your health:

PLACE
& address

NAMES
include people
you traveled with

describe the
social distancing

mask on others yes no

Arrival time

Departure time

washed hands before yes no

hand sanitizer before yes no

mask on you yes no

transportation

body temperature

outdoors or inside

# of people

washed hands after yes no

hand sanitizer after yes no

**DATE:**

**PLACE**
**& address**

**NAMES**
include people you traveled with

**mask on others** yes no

**Arrival time**

**Departure time**

**washed hands before** yes no

**hand sanitizer before** yes no

**mask on you** yes no

**transportation**

**body temperature**

**outdoors or inside**

**# of people**

**washed hands after** yes no

**hand sanitizer after** yes no

**your health:**

**describe the social distancing**

hand sanitizer after yes no

washed hands after yes no

# of people

outdoors or inside

body temperature

transportation

mask on you yes no

hand sanitizer before yes no

washed hands before yes no

Departure time

Arrival time

mask on others yes no

your health:

NAMES
include people you traveled with

PLACE
& address

describe the social distancing

DATE:

hand sanitizer after yes no

washed hands after yes no

# of people

outdoors or inside

body temperature

transportation

mask on you yes no

hand sanitizer before yes no

washed hands before yes no

Departure time

Arrival time

mask on others yes no

your health:

NAMES
include people you traveled with

PLACE
& address

describe the social distancing

DATE:

hand sanitizer after yes no

washed hands after yes no

# of people

outdoors or inside

body temperature

transportation

mask on you yes no

hand sanitizer before yes no

washed hands before yes no

**Departure time**

**Arrival time**

mask on others yes no

**your health:**

**NAMES** include people you traveled with

**PLACE** & address

**describe the social distancing**

**DATE:**

your health:

| PLACE & address | NAMES include people you traveled with | mask on others yes no | Arrival time | Departure time | washed hands before yes no | hand sanitizer before yes no | mask on you yes no | transportation | body temperature | outdoors or inside | # of people | washed hands after yes no | hand sanitizer after yes no |
|---|---|---|---|---|---|---|---|---|---|---|---|---|---|
| | describe the social distancing | | | | | | | | | | | | |



DATE:

DATE:

hand sanitizer after yes no

washed hands after yes no

# of people

outdoors or inside

body temperature

transportation

mask on you yes no

hand sanitizer before yes no

washed hands before yes no

**Departure time**

**Arrival time**

mask on others yes no

**PLACE** & address

**NAMES** include people you traveled with

your health:

describe the social distancing

hand sanitizer after yes no

washed hands after yes no

# of people

outdoors or inside

body temperature

transportation

mask on you yes no

hand sanitizer before yes no

washed hands before yes no

**Departure time**

**Arrival time**

mask on others yes no

**your health:**

**PLACE**
& address

**NAMES**
include people you traveled with

**describe the social distancing**

**DATE:**

hand sanitizer after yes no

washed hands after yes no

# of people

outdoors or inside

body temperature

transportation

mask on you yes no

hand sanitizer before yes no

washed hands before yes no

Departure time

Arrival time

mask on others yes no

your health:

NAMES
include people you traveled with

PLACE
& address

describe the social distancing

DATE:

hand sanitizer after yes no

washed hands after yes no

# of people

outdoors or inside

body temperature

transportation

mask on you yes no

hand sanitizer before yes no

washed hands before yes no

Departure time

Arrival time

mask on others yes no

your health:

PLACE
& address

NAMES
include people you traveled with

describe the social distancing

DATE:

DATE:

hand sanitizer after yes no

washed hands after yes no

# of people

outdoors or inside

body temperature

transportation

mask on you yes no

hand sanitizer before yes no

washed hands before yes no

Departure time

Arrival time

mask on others yes no

describe the social distancing

NAMES include people you traveled with

PLACE & address

your health:

hand sanitizer after yes no

washed hands after yes no

# of people

outdoors or inside

body temperature

transportation

mask on you yes no

hand sanitizer before yes no

washed hands before yes no

**Departure time**

**Arrival time**

mask on others yes no

your health:

**PLACE** & address

**NAMES** include people you traveled with

describe the social distancing

DATE:

hand sanitizer after yes no

washed hands after yes no

# of people

outdoors or inside

body temperature

transportation

mask on you yes no

hand sanitizer before yes no

washed hands before yes no

Departure time

Arrival time

mask on others yes no

your health:

NAMES include people you traveled with

PLACE & address

describe the social distancing

DATE:

hand sanitizer after yes no

washed hands after yes no

# of people

outdoors or inside

body temperature

transportation

mask on you yes no

hand sanitizer before yes no

washed hands before yes no

Departure time

Arrival time

mask on others yes no

your health:

**PLACE**
& address

**NAMES**
include people you traveled with

describe the social distancing

**DATE:**

hand sanitizer after yes no

washed hands after yes no

# of people

outdoors or inside

body temperature

transportation

mask on you yes no

hand sanitizer before yes no

washed hands before yes no

Departure time

Arrival time

mask on others yes no

your health:

NAMES
include people you traveled with

PLACE
& address

describe the social distancing

DATE:

hand sanitizer after yes no

washed hands after yes no

# of people

outdoors or inside

body temperature

transportation

mask on you yes no

hand sanitizer before yes no

washed hands before yes no

**Departure time**

**Arrival time**

mask on others yes no

**DATE:**

**your health:**

**PLACE**
& address

**NAMES**
include people you traveled with

**describe the social distancing**

hand sanitizer after yes no

washed hands after yes no

# of people

outdoors or inside

body temperature

transportation

mask on you yes no

hand sanitizer before yes no

washed hands before yes no

Departure time

Arrival time

mask on others yes no

your health:

**NAMES**
include people you traveled with

**PLACE**
& address

describe the social distancing

DATE:

DATE:

hand sanitizer after yes no

washed hands after yes no

# of people

outdoors or inside

body temperature

transportation

mask on you yes no

hand sanitizer before yes no

washed hands before yes no

Departure time

Arrival time

mask on others yes no

**your health:**

**PLACE** & address

**NAMES** include people you traveled with

describe the social distancing

PLACE
& address

NAMES
include people
you traveled with

your health:

mask on others yes no

Arrival time

Departure time

washed hands before yes no

hand sanitizer before yes no

mask on you yes no

transportation

body temperature

outdoors or inside

# of people

washed hands after yes no

hand sanitizer after yes no

describe the
social distancing

DATE:

DATE:

hand sanitizer after yes no

washed hands after yes no

# of people

outdoors or inside

body temperature

transportation

mask on you yes no

hand sanitizer before yes no

washed hands before yes no

**Departure time**

**Arrival time**

mask on others yes no

your health:

**NAMES**
include people you traveled with

**PLACE**
& address

describe the social distancing

DATE:

your health:

PLACE
& address

NAMES
include people
you traveled with

describe the
social distancing

mask on others yes no

Arrival time

Departure time

washed hands before yes no

hand sanitizer before yes no

mask on you yes no

transportation

body temperature

outdoors or inside

# of people

washed hands after yes no

hand sanitizer after yes no

DATE:

hand sanitizer after yes no

washed hands after yes no

# of people

outdoors or inside

body temperature

transportation

mask on you yes no

hand sanitizer before yes no

washed hands before yes no

Departure time

Arrival time

mask on others yes no

your health:

**PLACE**
& address

**NAMES**
include people you traveled with

describe the social distancing

DATE:

your health:

**PLACE**
& address

**NAMES**
include people
you traveled with

mask on others yes no

**Arrival time**

**Departure time**

washed hands before yes no

hand sanitizer before yes no

mask on you yes no

transportation

body temperature

outdoors or inside

# of people

washed hands after yes no

hand sanitizer after yes no

describe the
social distancing

your health:

| PLACE & address | NAMES include people you traveled with | mask on others yes no | Arrival time | Departure time | washed hands before yes no | hand sanitizer before yes no | mask on you yes no | transportation | body temperature | outdoors or inside | # of people | washed hands after yes no | hand sanitizer after yes no |
|---|---|---|---|---|---|---|---|---|---|---|---|---|---|
| | describe the social distancing | | | | | | | | | | | | |



DATE:

hand sanitizer after yes no

washed hands after yes no

# of people

outdoors or inside

body temperature

transportation

mask on you yes no

hand sanitizer before yes no

washed hands before yes no

Departure time

Arrival time

mask on others yes no

NAMES include people you traveled with

describe the social distancing

PLACE & address

your health:

DATE:

DATE:

hand sanitizer after yes no

washed hands after yes no

# of people

outdoors or inside

body temperature

transportation

mask on you yes no

hand sanitizer before yes no

washed hands before yes no

Departure time

Arrival time

mask on others yes no

your health:

PLACE & address

NAMES include people you traveled with

describe the social distancing

your health:

| PLACE & address | NAMES include people you traveled with | mask on others yes no | Arrival time | Departure time | washed hands before yes no | hand sanitizer before yes no | mask on you yes no | transportation | body temperature | outdoors or inside | # of people | washed hands after yes no | hand sanitizer after yes no |
|---|---|---|---|---|---|---|---|---|---|---|---|---|---|
| | describe the social distancing | | | | | | | | | | | | |



DATE:

hand sanitizer after yes no

washed hands after yes no

# of people

outdoors or inside

body temperature

transportation

mask on you yes no

hand sanitizer before yes no

washed hands before yes no

**Departure time**

**Arrival time**

mask on others yes no

**DATE:**

**your health:**

**PLACE** & address

**NAMES** include people you traveled with

describe the social distancing

DATE:

your health:

**PLACE** & address

**NAMES** include people you traveled with

describe the social distancing

mask on others yes no

**Arrival time**

**Departure time**

washed hands before yes no

hand sanitizer before yes no

mask on you yes no

transportation

body temperature

outdoors or inside

# of people

washed hands after yes no

hand sanitizer after yes no

DATE:

hand sanitizer after yes no

washed hands after yes no

# of people

outdoors or inside

body temperature

transportation

mask on you yes no

hand sanitizer before yes no

washed hands before yes no

**Departure time**

**Arrival time**

mask on others yes no

**NAMES** include people you traveled with

**PLACE** & address

your health:

describe the social distancing

hand sanitizer after yes no

washed hands after yes no

# of people

outdoors or inside

body temperature

transportation

mask on you yes no

hand sanitizer before yes no

washed hands before yes no

Departure time

Arrival time

mask on others yes no

DATE:

your health:

**NAMES** include people you traveled with

**PLACE** & address

describe the social distancing

DATE:

your health:

**PLACE** & address

**NAMES** include people you traveled with

describe the social distancing

mask on others yes no

**Arrival time**

**Departure time**

washed hands before yes no

hand sanitizer before yes no

mask on you yes no

transportation

body temperature

outdoors or inside

# of people

washed hands after yes no

hand sanitizer after yes no

your health:

**PLACE** & address

**NAMES** include people you traveled with

mask on others yes no

**Arrival time**

**Departure time**

washed hands before yes no

hand sanitizer before yes no

mask on you yes no

transportation

body temperature

outdoors or inside

# of people

washed hands after yes no

hand sanitizer after yes no

describe the social distancing

**DATE:**

hand sanitizer after yes no

washed hands after yes no

# of people

outdoors or inside

body temperature

transportation

mask on you yes no

hand sanitizer before yes no

washed hands before yes no

**Departure time**

**Arrival time**

mask on others yes no

**your health:**

**NAMES**
include people you traveled with

**PLACE**
& address

**describe the social distancing**

**DATE:**

your health:

| PLACE & address | NAMES include people you traveled with | mask on others yes no | Arrival time | Departure time | washed hands before yes no | hand sanitizer before yes no | mask on you yes no | transportation | body temperature | outdoors or inside | # of people | washed hands after yes no | hand sanitizer after yes no |
|---|---|---|---|---|---|---|---|---|---|---|---|---|---|
| | describe the social distancing | | | | | | | | | | | | |



DATE:

hand sanitizer after yes no

washed hands after yes no

# of people

outdoors or inside

body temperature

transportation

mask on you yes no

hand sanitizer before yes no

washed hands before yes no

Departure time

Arrival time

mask on others yes no

your health:

NAMES include people you traveled with

PLACE & address

describe the social distancing

DATE:

hand sanitizer after yes no

washed hands after yes no

# of people

outdoors or inside

body temperature

transportation

mask on you yes no

hand sanitizer before yes no

washed hands before yes no

Departure time

Arrival time

mask on others yes no

DATE:

your health:

PLACE
& address

NAMES
include people you traveled with

describe the social distancing

hand sanitizer after yes no

washed hands after yes no

# of people

outdoors or inside

body temperature

transportation

mask on you yes no

hand sanitizer before yes no

washed hands before yes no

Departure time

Arrival time

mask on others yes no

your health:

PLACE
& address

NAMES
include people you traveled with

describe the social distancing

DATE:

DATE:

your health:

PLACE
& address

NAMES
include people
you traveled with

mask on others yes no

Arrival time

Departure time

washed hands before yes no

hand sanitizer before yes no

mask on you yes no

transportation

body temperature

outdoors or inside

# of people

washed hands after yes no

hand sanitizer after yes no

describe the
social distancing

DATE:

hand sanitizer after yes no

washed hands after yes no

# of people

outdoors or inside

body temperature

transportation

mask on you yes no

hand sanitizer before yes no

washed hands before yes no

**Departure time**

**Arrival time**

mask on others yes no

**PLACE** & address

**NAMES** include people you traveled with

describe the social distancing

your health:

hand sanitizer after yes no

washed hands after yes no

# of people

outdoors or inside

body temperature

transportation

mask on you yes no

hand sanitizer before yes no

washed hands before yes no

Departure time

Arrival time

mask on others yes no

your health:

PLACE & address

NAMES include people you traveled with

describe the social distancing

DATE:

DATE:

your health:

PLACE
& address

NAMES
include people you traveled with

describe the social distancing

mask on others yes no

Arrival time

Departure time

washed hands before yes no

hand sanitizer before yes no

mask on you yes no

transportation

body temperature

outdoors or inside

# of people

washed hands after yes no

hand sanitizer after yes no

hand sanitizer after yes no

washed hands after yes no

# of people

outdoors or inside

body temperature

transportation

mask on you yes no

hand sanitizer before yes no

washed hands before yes no

**Departure time**

**Arrival time**

mask on others yes no

**DATE:**

**your health:**

**NAMES** include people you traveled with

**PLACE** & address

**describe the social distancing**

hand sanitizer after yes no

washed hands after yes no

# of people

outdoors or inside

body temperature

transportation

mask on you yes no

hand sanitizer before yes no

washed hands before yes no

Departure time

Arrival time

mask on others yes no

your health:

**NAMES** include people you traveled with

**PLACE** & address

describe the social distancing

**DATE:**

DATE:

your health:

**PLACE**
& address

**NAMES**
include people you traveled with

describe the social distancing

mask on others yes no

**Arrival time**

**Departure time**

washed hands before yes no

hand sanitizer before yes no

mask on you yes no

transportation

body temperature

outdoors or inside

# of people

washed hands after yes no

hand sanitizer after yes no

your health:

| PLACE & address | NAMES include people you traveled with | mask on others yes no | Arrival time | Departure time | washed hands before yes no | hand sanitizer before yes no | mask on you yes no | transportation | body temperature | outdoors or inside | # of people | washed hands after yes no | hand sanitizer after yes no |
|---|---|---|---|---|---|---|---|---|---|---|---|---|---|
| | describe the social distancing | | | | | | | | | | | | |



DATE:

DATE:

hand sanitizer after yes no

washed hands after yes no

# of people

outdoors or inside

body temperature

transportation

mask on you yes no

hand sanitizer before yes no

washed hands before yes no

Departure time

Arrival time

mask on others yes no

describe the social distancing

NAMES include people you traveled with

PLACE & address

your health:

DATE:

hand sanitizer after yes no

washed hands after yes no

# of people

outdoors or inside

body temperature

transportation

mask on you yes no

hand sanitizer before yes no

washed hands before yes no

Departure time

Arrival time

mask on others yes no

your health:

PLACE & address

NAMES include people you traveled with

describe the social distancing

hand sanitizer after yes no

washed hands after yes no

# of people

outdoors or inside

body temperature

transportation

mask on you yes no

hand sanitizer before yes no

washed hands before yes no

Departure time

Arrival time

mask on others yes no

your health:

NAMES
include people you traveled with

PLACE
& address

describe the social distancing

DATE:

hand sanitizer after yes no

washed hands after yes no

# of people

outdoors or inside

body temperature

transportation

mask on you yes no

hand sanitizer before yes no

washed hands before yes no

Departure time

Arrival time

mask on others yes no

DATE:

your health:

PLACE & address

NAMES include people you traveled with

describe the social distancing

DATE:

hand sanitizer after yes no

washed hands after yes no

# of people

outdoors or inside

body temperature

transportation

mask on you yes no

hand sanitizer before yes no

washed hands before yes no

**Departure time**

**Arrival time**

mask on others yes no

describe the social distancing

**NAMES**
include people you traveled with

**PLACE**
& address

your health:

hand sanitizer after yes no

washed hands after yes no

# of people

outdoors or inside

body temperature

transportation

mask on you yes no

hand sanitizer before yes no

washed hands before yes no

Departure time

Arrival time

mask on others yes no

your health:

PLACE & address

NAMES include people you traveled with

describe the social distancing

DATE:

DATE:

hand sanitizer after yes no

washed hands after yes no

# of people

outdoors or inside

body temperature

transportation

mask on you yes no

hand sanitizer before yes no

washed hands before yes no

**Departure time**

**Arrival time**

mask on others yes no

**PLACE**
& address

**NAMES**
include people you traveled with

your health:

describe the social distancing

hand sanitizer after yes no

washed hands after yes no

# of people

outdoors or inside

body temperature

transportation

mask on you yes no

hand sanitizer before yes no

washed hands before yes no

**Departure time**

**Arrival time**

mask on others yes no

your health:

**PLACE**
& address

**NAMES**
include people you traveled with

describe the social distancing

**DATE:**

DATE:

hand sanitizer after yes no

washed hands after yes no

# of people

outdoors or inside

body temperature

transportation

mask on you yes no

hand sanitizer before yes no

washed hands before yes no

Departure time

Arrival time

mask on others yes no

NAMES
include people you traveled with

PLACE
& address

your health:

describe the social distancing

**DATE:**

hand sanitizer after yes no

washed hands after yes no

# of people

outdoors or inside

body temperature

transportation

mask on you yes no

hand sanitizer before yes no

washed hands before yes no

**Departure time**

**Arrival time**

mask on others yes no

**your health:**

**PLACE**
& address

**NAMES**
include people you traveled with

**describe the social distancing**

hand sanitizer after yes no

washed hands after yes no

# of people

outdoors or inside

body temperature

transportation

mask on you yes no

hand sanitizer before yes no

washed hands before yes no

**Departure time**

**Arrival time**

mask on others yes no

your health:

**NAMES**
include people you traveled with

**PLACE**
& address

describe the social distancing

**DATE:**

DATE:

your health:

PLACE
& address

NAMES
include people
you traveled with

describe the
social distancing

| | |
|---|---|
| hand sanitizer after | yes no |
| washed hands after | yes no |
| # of people | |
| outdoors or inside | |
| body temperature | |
| transportation | |
| mask on you | yes no |
| hand sanitizer before | yes no |
| washed hands before | yes no |
| Departure time | |
| Arrival time | |
| mask on others | yes no |

hand sanitizer after yes no

washed hands after yes no

# of people

outdoors or inside

body temperature

transportation

mask on you yes no

hand sanitizer before yes no

washed hands before yes no

**Departure time**

**Arrival time**

mask on others yes no

describe the social distancing

**NAMES** include people you traveled with

**PLACE** & address

your health:

**DATE:**

DATE:

your health:

**PLACE**
& address

**NAMES**
include people you traveled with

mask on others yes no

**Arrival time**

**Departure time**

washed hands before yes no

hand sanitizer before yes no

mask on you yes no

transportation

body temperature

outdoors or inside

# of people

washed hands after yes no

hand sanitizer after yes no

describe the social distancing

hand sanitizer after yes no

washed hands after yes no

# of people

outdoors or inside

body temperature

transportation

mask on you yes no

hand sanitizer before yes no

washed hands before yes no

Departure time

Arrival time

mask on others yes no

DATE:

your health:

**NAMES** include people you traveled with

**PLACE** & address

describe the social distancing

hand sanitizer after yes no

washed hands after yes no

# of people

outdoors or inside

body temperature

transportation

mask on you yes no

hand sanitizer before yes no

washed hands before yes no

Departure time

Arrival time

mask on others yes no

your health:

NAMES include people you traveled with

PLACE & address

describe the social distancing

DATE:

hand sanitizer after yes no

washed hands after yes no

# of people

outdoors or inside

body temperature

transportation

mask on you yes no

hand sanitizer before yes no

washed hands before yes no

Departure time

Arrival time

mask on others yes no

**DATE:**

your health:

**NAMES**
include people you traveled with

**PLACE**
& address

describe the social distancing

DATE:

hand sanitizer after yes no

washed hands after yes no

# of people

outdoors or inside

body temperature

transportation

mask on you yes no

hand sanitizer before yes no

washed hands before yes no

**Departure time**

**Arrival time**

mask on others yes no

**NAMES** include people you traveled with

**PLACE** & address

your health:

describe the social distancing

your health:

| PLACE & address | NAMES include people you traveled with | mask on others yes no | Arrival time | Departure time | washed hands before yes no | hand sanitizer before yes no | mask on you yes no | transportation | body temperature | outdoors or inside | # of people | washed hands after yes no | hand sanitizer after yes no |
|---|---|---|---|---|---|---|---|---|---|---|---|---|---|
| | describe the social distancing | | | | | | | | | | | | |



DATE:

hand sanitizer after yes no

washed hands after yes no

# of people

outdoors or inside

body temperature

transportation

mask on you yes no

hand sanitizer before yes no

washed hands before yes no

Departure time

Arrival time

mask on others yes no

your health:

**PLACE**
& address

**NAMES**
include people you traveled with

**describe the social distancing**

**DATE:**

your health:

| PLACE & address | NAMES include people you traveled with | mask on others yes no | Arrival time | Departure time | washed hands before yes no | hand sanitizer before yes no | mask on you yes no | transportation | body temperature | outdoors or inside | # of people | washed hands after yes no | hand sanitizer after yes no |
|---|---|---|---|---|---|---|---|---|---|---|---|---|---|
| | describe the social distancing | | | | | | | | | | | | |



DATE:

DATE:

**PLACE** & address

**NAMES** include people you traveled with

your health:

mask on others yes no

**Arrival time**

**Departure time**

washed hands before yes no

hand sanitizer before yes no

mask on you yes no

transportation

body temperature

outdoors or inside

# of people

washed hands after yes no

hand sanitizer after yes no

describe the social distancing

your health:

| PLACE & address | NAMES include people you traveled with | mask on others yes no | Arrival time | Departure time | washed hands before yes no | hand sanitizer before yes no | mask on you yes no | transportation | body temperature | outdoors or inside | # of people | washed hands after yes no | hand sanitizer after yes no |
|---|---|---|---|---|---|---|---|---|---|---|---|---|---|

describe the social distancing



DATE:

hand sanitizer after yes no

washed hands after yes no

# of people

outdoors or inside

body temperature

transportation

mask on you yes no

hand sanitizer before yes no

washed hands before yes no

Departure time

Arrival time

mask on others yes no

DATE:

your health:

NAMES
include people you traveled with

PLACE
& address

describe the social distancing

your health:

| PLACE & address | NAMES include people you traveled with | mask on others yes no | Arrival time | Departure time | washed hands before yes no | hand sanitizer before yes no | mask on you yes no | transportation | body temperature | outdoors or inside | # of people | washed hands after yes no | hand sanitizer after yes no |
|---|---|---|---|---|---|---|---|---|---|---|---|---|---|
| | | | | | | | | | | | | | |

describe the social distancing



DATE:

DATE:

PLACE
& address

NAMES
include people
you traveled with

mask on others yes no

Arrival time

Departure time

washed hands before yes no

hand sanitizer before yes no

mask on you yes no

transportation

body temperature

outdoors or inside

# of people

washed hands after yes no

hand sanitizer after yes no

your health:

describe the
social distancing

**DATE:**

| PLACE & address | NAMES include people you traveled with | mask on others yes no | Arrival time | Departure time | washed hands before yes no | hand sanitizer before yes no | mask on you yes no | transportation | body temperature | outdoors or inside | # of people | washed hands after yes no | hand sanitizer after yes no |
|---|---|---|---|---|---|---|---|---|---|---|---|---|---|
| | | | | | | | | | | | | | |

describe the social distancing

your health:

hand sanitizer after yes no

washed hands after yes no

# of people

outdoors or inside

body temperature

transportation

mask on you yes no

hand sanitizer before yes no

washed hands before yes no

Departure time

Arrival time

mask on others yes no

DATE:

your health:

NAMES
include people you traveled with

PLACE
& address

describe the social distancing

your health:

| PLACE & address | NAMES include people you traveled with | mask on others yes no | Arrival time | Departure time | washed hands before yes no | hand sanitizer before yes no | mask on you yes no | transportation | body temperature | outdoors or inside | # of people | washed hands after yes no | hand sanitizer after yes no |
|---|---|---|---|---|---|---|---|---|---|---|---|---|---|
| | describe the social distancing | | | | | | | | | | | | |



DATE:

DATE:

hand sanitizer after yes no

washed hands after yes no

# of people

outdoors or inside

body temperature

transportation

mask on you yes no

hand sanitizer before yes no

washed hands before yes no

Departure time

Arrival time

mask on others yes no

your health:

NAMES include people you traveled with

PLACE & address

describe the social distancing

hand sanitizer after yes no

washed hands after yes no

# of people

outdoors or inside

body temperature

transportation

mask on you yes no

hand sanitizer before yes no

washed hands before yes no

**Departure time**

**Arrival time**

mask on others yes no

**your health:**

**PLACE**
& address

**NAMES**
include people you traveled with

describe the social distancing

**DATE:**

hand sanitizer after yes no

washed hands after yes no

# of people

outdoors or inside

body temperature

transportation

mask on you yes no

hand sanitizer before yes no

washed hands before yes no

Departure time

Arrival time

mask on others yes no

DATE:

PLACE & address

NAMES include people you traveled with

describe the social distancing

your health:

your health:

| PLACE & address | NAMES include people you traveled with | mask on others yes no | Arrival time | Departure time | washed hands before yes no | hand sanitizer before yes no | mask on you yes no | transportation | body temperature | outdoors or inside | # of people | washed hands after yes no | hand sanitizer after yes no |
|---|---|---|---|---|---|---|---|---|---|---|---|---|---|
| | | | | | | | | | | | | | |

describe the social distancing



DATE:

hand sanitizer after yes no

washed hands after yes no

# of people

outdoors or inside

body temperature

transportation

mask on you yes no

hand sanitizer before yes no

washed hands before yes no

Departure time

Arrival time

mask on others yes no

DATE:

your health:

NAMES
include people you traveled with

PLACE
& address

describe the social distancing

DATE:

your health:

PLACE
& address

NAMES
include people
you traveled with

mask on others yes no

Arrival time

Departure time

washed hands before yes no

hand sanitizer before yes no

mask on you yes no

transportation

body temperature

outdoors or inside

# of people

washed hands after yes no

hand sanitizer after yes no

describe the
social distancing

your health:

| PLACE & address | NAMES include people you traveled with | mask on others yes no | Arrival time | Departure time | washed hands before yes no | hand sanitizer before yes no | mask on you yes no | transportation | body temperature | outdoors or inside | # of people | washed hands after yes no | hand sanitizer after yes no |
|---|---|---|---|---|---|---|---|---|---|---|---|---|---|
| | describe the social distancing | | | | | | | | | | | | |



DATE:

your health:

| PLACE & address | NAMES include people you traveled with | mask on others yes no | Arrival time | Departure time | washed hands before yes no | hand sanitizer before yes no | mask on you yes no | transportation | body temperature | outdoors or inside | # of people | washed hands after yes no | hand sanitizer after yes no |
|---|---|---|---|---|---|---|---|---|---|---|---|---|---|

describe the social distancing



DATE:

DATE:

hand sanitizer after yes no

washed hands after yes no

# of people

outdoors or inside

body temperature

transportation

mask on you yes no

hand sanitizer before yes no

washed hands before yes no

**Departure time**

**Arrival time**

mask on others yes no

your health:

**PLACE** & address

**NAMES** include people you traveled with

describe the social distancing

your health:

| PLACE & address | NAMES include people you traveled with | mask on others yes no | Arrival time | Departure time | washed hands before yes no | hand sanitizer before yes no | mask on you yes no | transportation | body temperature | outdoors or inside | # of people | washed hands after yes no | hand sanitizer after yes no |
|---|---|---|---|---|---|---|---|---|---|---|---|---|---|
| | | | | | | | | | | | | | |

describe the social distancing



DATE:

DATE:

your health:

PLACE
& address

NAMES
include people
you traveled with

describe the
social distancing

mask on others yes no

Arrival time

Departure time

washed hands before yes no

hand sanitizer before yes no

mask on you yes no

transportation

body temperature

outdoors or inside

# of people

washed hands after yes no

hand sanitizer after yes no

your health:

| PLACE & address | NAMES include people you traveled with | mask on others yes no | Arrival time | Departure time | washed hands before yes no | hand sanitizer before yes no | mask on you yes no | transportation | body temperature | outdoors or inside | # of people | washed hands after yes no | hand sanitizer after yes no |
|---|---|---|---|---|---|---|---|---|---|---|---|---|---|
| | | | | | | | | | | | | | |

describe the social distancing



DATE:

hand sanitizer after yes no

washed hands after yes no

# of people

outdoors or inside

body temperature

transportation

mask on you yes no

hand sanitizer before yes no

washed hands before yes no

**Departure time**

**Arrival time**

mask on others yes no

**DATE:**

**your health:**

**PLACE** & address

**NAMES** include people you traveled with

describe the social distancing

your health:

| PLACE & address | NAMES include people you traveled with | mask on others yes no | Arrival time | Departure time | washed hands before yes no | hand sanitizer before yes no | mask on you yes no | transportation | body temperature | outdoors or inside | # of people | washed hands after yes no | hand sanitizer after yes no |
|---|---|---|---|---|---|---|---|---|---|---|---|---|---|
| | | | | | | | | | | | | | |

describe the social distancing



DATE:

hand sanitizer after yes no

washed hands after yes no

# of people

outdoors or inside

body temperature

transportation

mask on you yes no

hand sanitizer before yes no

washed hands before yes no

**Departure time**

**Arrival time**

mask on others yes no

**your health:**

**NAMES** include people you traveled with

**PLACE** & address

describe the social distancing

**DATE:**

DATE:

**PLACE**
& address

**NAMES**
include people you traveled with

your health:

mask on others yes no

**Arrival time**

**Departure time**

washed hands before yes no

hand sanitizer before yes no

mask on you yes no

transportation

body temperature

outdoors or inside

# of people

washed hands after yes no

hand sanitizer after yes no

describe the social distancing

DATE:

hand sanitizer after yes no

washed hands after yes no

# of people

outdoors or inside

body temperature

transportation

mask on you yes no

hand sanitizer before yes no

washed hands before yes no

Departure time

Arrival time

mask on others yes no

describe the social distancing

NAMES
include people you traveled with

PLACE
& address

your health:

hand sanitizer after yes no

washed hands after yes no

# of people

outdoors or inside

body temperature

transportation

mask on you yes no

hand sanitizer before yes no

washed hands before yes no

Departure time

Arrival time

mask on others yes no

DATE:

your health:

NAMES include people you traveled with

PLACE & address

describe the social distancing

DATE:

hand sanitizer after yes no

washed hands after yes no

# of people

outdoors or inside

body temperature

transportation

mask on you yes no

hand sanitizer before yes no

washed hands before yes no

**Departure time**

**Arrival time**

mask on others yes no

**PLACE** & address

**NAMES** include people you traveled with

describe the social distancing

your health:

hand sanitizer after yes no

washed hands after yes no

# of people

outdoors or inside

body temperature

transportation

mask on you yes no

hand sanitizer before yes no

washed hands before yes no

Departure time

Arrival time

mask on others yes no

your health:

**PLACE**
& address

**NAMES**
include people you traveled with

describe the social distancing

DATE:

hand sanitizer after yes no

washed hands after yes no

# of people

outdoors or inside

body temperature

transportation

mask on you yes no

hand sanitizer before yes no

washed hands before yes no

Departure time

Arrival time

mask on others yes no

DATE:

your health:

**PLACE**
& address

**NAMES**
include people you traveled with

describe the social distancing

hand sanitizer after yes no

washed hands after yes no

# of people

outdoors or inside

body temperature

transportation

mask on you yes no

hand sanitizer before yes no

washed hands before yes no

**Departure time**

**Arrival time**

mask on others yes no

your health:

**NAMES**
include people you traveled with

**PLACE**
& address

describe the social distancing

DATE:

hand sanitizer after yes no

washed hands after yes no

# of people

outdoors or inside

body temperature

transportation

mask on you yes no

hand sanitizer before yes no

washed hands before yes no

**Departure time**

**Arrival time**

mask on others yes no

**NAMES**
include people you traveled with

**PLACE**
& address

your health:

describe the social distancing

**DATE:**

your health:

| PLACE & address | NAMES include people you traveled with | mask on others yes no | Arrival time | Departure time | washed hands before yes no | hand sanitizer before yes no | mask on you yes no | transportation | body temperature | outdoors or inside | # of people | washed hands after yes no | hand sanitizer after yes no |
|---|---|---|---|---|---|---|---|---|---|---|---|---|---|
| | | | | | | | | | | | | | |

describe the social distancing



DATE:

hand sanitizer after yes no

washed hands after yes no

# of people

outdoors or inside

body temperature

transportation

mask on you yes no

hand sanitizer before yes no

washed hands before yes no

Departure time

Arrival time

mask on others yes no

DATE:

your health:

NAMES include people you traveled with

PLACE & address

describe the social distancing

DATE:

PLACE
& address

NAMES
include people
you traveled with

mask on others yes no

Arrival time

Departure time

washed hands before yes no

hand sanitizer before yes no

mask on you yes no

transportation

body temperature

outdoors or inside

# of people

washed hands after yes no

hand sanitizer after yes no

your health:

describe the
social distancing

DATE:

your health:

PLACE
& address

NAMES
include people
you traveled with

describe the
social distancing

mask on others yes no

Arrival time

Departure time

washed hands before yes no

hand sanitizer before yes no

mask on you yes no

transportation

body temperature

outdoors or inside

# of people

washed hands after yes no

hand sanitizer after yes no

hand sanitizer after yes no

washed hands after yes no

# of people

outdoors or inside

body temperature

transportation

mask on you yes no

hand sanitizer before yes no

washed hands before yes no

Departure time

Arrival time

mask on others yes no

DATE:

PLACE & address

NAMES include people you traveled with

your health:

describe the social distancing

**DATE:**

hand sanitizer after yes no

washed hands after yes no

# of people

outdoors or inside

body temperature

transportation

mask on you yes no

hand sanitizer before yes no

washed hands before yes no

**Departure time**

**Arrival time**

mask on others yes no

**describe the social distancing**

**NAMES** include people you traveled with

**PLACE** & address

**your health:**

hand sanitizer after yes no

washed hands after yes no

# of people

outdoors or inside

body temperature

transportation

mask on you yes no

hand sanitizer before yes no

washed hands before yes no

**Departure time**

**Arrival time**

mask on others yes no

**NAMES** include people you traveled with

**PLACE** & address

**your health:**

**describe the social distancing**

**DATE:**

DATE:

hand sanitizer after yes no

washed hands after yes no

# of people

outdoors or inside

body temperature

transportation

mask on you yes no

hand sanitizer before yes no

washed hands before yes no

**Departure time**

**Arrival time**

mask on others yes no

your health:

**NAMES** include people you traveled with

**PLACE** & address

describe the social distancing

your health:

| PLACE & address | NAMES include people you traveled with | mask on others yes no | Arrival time | Departure time | washed hands before yes no | hand sanitizer before yes no | mask on you yes no | transportation | body temperature | outdoors or inside | # of people | washed hands after yes no | hand sanitizer after yes no |
|---|---|---|---|---|---|---|---|---|---|---|---|---|---|
| | | | | | | | | | | | | | |

describe the social distancing



DATE:

hand sanitizer after yes no

washed hands after yes no

# of people

outdoors or inside

body temperature

transportation

mask on you yes no

hand sanitizer before yes no

washed hands before yes no

Departure time

Arrival time

mask on others yes no

your health:

**NAMES** include people you traveled with

**PLACE** & address

describe the social distancing

**DATE:**

your health:

| PLACE & address | NAMES include people you traveled with | mask on others yes no | Arrival time | Departure time | washed hands before yes no | hand sanitizer before yes no | mask on you yes no | transportation | body temperature | outdoors or inside | # of people | washed hands after yes no | hand sanitizer after yes no |
|---|---|---|---|---|---|---|---|---|---|---|---|---|---|
| | describe the social distancing | | | | | | | | | | | | |



DATE:

DATE:

your health:

PLACE
& address

NAMES
include people
you traveled with

describe the
social distancing

mask on others yes no

Arrival time

Departure time

washed hands before yes no

hand sanitizer before yes no

mask on you yes no

transportation

body temperature

outdoors or inside

# of people

washed hands after yes no

hand sanitizer after yes no

DATE:

your health:

PLACE
& address

NAMES
include people you traveled with

mask on others yes no

Arrival time

Departure time

washed hands before yes no

hand sanitizer before yes no

mask on you yes no

transportation

body temperature

outdoors or inside

# of people

washed hands after yes no

hand sanitizer after yes no

describe the social distancing

DATE:

hand sanitizer after yes no

washed hands after yes no

# of people

outdoors or inside

body temperature

transportation

mask on you yes no

hand sanitizer before yes no

washed hands before yes no

**Departure time**

**Arrival time**

mask on others yes no

describe the social distancing

**NAMES** include people you traveled with

**PLACE** & address

your health:

your health:

| PLACE & address | NAMES include people you traveled with | mask on others yes no | Arrival time | Departure time | washed hands before yes no | hand sanitizer before yes no | mask on you yes no | transportation | body temperature | outdoors or inside | # of people | washed hands after yes no | hand sanitizer after yes no |
|---|---|---|---|---|---|---|---|---|---|---|---|---|---|
| | | | | | | | | | | | | | |

describe the social distancing



DATE:

DATE:

your health:

PLACE
& address

NAMES
include people
you traveled with

mask on others yes no

Arrival time

Departure time

washed hands before yes no

hand sanitizer before yes no

mask on you yes no

transportation

body temperature

outdoors or inside

# of people

washed hands after yes no

hand sanitizer after yes no

describe the
social distancing

hand sanitizer after yes no

washed hands after yes no

# of people

outdoors or inside

body temperature

transportation

mask on you yes no

hand sanitizer before yes no

washed hands before yes no

Departure time

Arrival time

mask on others yes no

NAMES include people you traveled with

PLACE & address

your health:

describe the social distancing

DATE:

hand sanitizer after yes no

washed hands after yes no

# of people

outdoors or inside

body temperature

transportation

mask on you yes no

hand sanitizer before yes no

washed hands before yes no

**Departure time**

**Arrival time**

mask on others yes no

your health:

**NAMES** include people you traveled with

**PLACE** & address

describe the social distancing

**DATE:**

your health:

| PLACE & address | NAMES include people you traveled with | mask on others yes no | Arrival time | Departure time | washed hands before yes no | hand sanitizer before yes no | mask on you yes no | transportation | body temperature | outdoors or inside | # of people | washed hands after yes no | hand sanitizer after yes no |
|---|---|---|---|---|---|---|---|---|---|---|---|---|---|
| | | | | | | | | | | | | | |

describe the social distancing



DATE:

hand sanitizer after yes no

washed hands after yes no

# of people

outdoors or inside

body temperature

transportation

mask on you yes no

hand sanitizer before yes no

washed hands before yes no

Departure time

Arrival time

mask on others yes no

your health:

NAMES
include people you traveled with

PLACE
& address

describe the social distancing

DATE:

your health:

| PLACE & address | NAMES include people you traveled with | mask on others yes no | Arrival time | Departure time | washed hands before yes no | hand sanitizer before yes no | mask on you yes no | transportation | body temperature | outdoors or inside | # of people | washed hands after yes no | hand sanitizer after yes no |
|---|---|---|---|---|---|---|---|---|---|---|---|---|---|
| | | | | | | | | | | | | | |

describe the social distancing



DATE:

hand sanitizer after yes no

washed hands after yes no

# of people

outdoors or inside

body temperature

transportation

mask on you yes no

hand sanitizer before yes no

washed hands before yes no

Departure time

Arrival time

mask on others yes no

DATE:

describe the social distancing

your health:

NAMES
include people you traveled with

PLACE
& address

your health:

| PLACE & address | NAMES include people you traveled with | mask on others yes no | Arrival time | Departure time | washed hands before yes no | hand sanitizer before yes no | mask on you yes no | transportation | body temperature | outdoors or inside | # of people | washed hands after yes no | hand sanitizer after yes no |
|---|---|---|---|---|---|---|---|---|---|---|---|---|---|
| | describe the social distancing | | | | | | | | | | | | |



DATE:

hand sanitizer after yes no

washed hands after yes no

# of people

outdoors or inside

body temperature

transportation

mask on you yes no

hand sanitizer before yes no

washed hands before yes no

Departure time

Arrival time

mask on others yes no

your health:

NAMES include people you traveled with

PLACE & address

describe the social distancing

DATE:

your health:

| PLACE & address | NAMES include people you traveled with | mask on others yes no | Arrival time | Departure time | washed hands before yes no | hand sanitizer before yes no | mask on you yes no | transportation | body temperature | outdoors or inside | # of people | washed hands after yes no | hand sanitizer after yes no |
|---|---|---|---|---|---|---|---|---|---|---|---|---|---|
| | | | | | | | | | | | | | |

describe the social distancing



DATE:

DATE:

PLACE & address

NAMES include people you traveled with

your health:

mask on others yes no

Arrival time

Departure time

washed hands before yes no

hand sanitizer before yes no

mask on you yes no

transportation

body temperature

outdoors or inside

# of people

washed hands after yes no

hand sanitizer after yes no

describe the social distancing

hand sanitizer after yes no

washed hands after yes no

# of people

outdoors or inside

body temperature

transportation

mask on you yes no

hand sanitizer before yes no

washed hands before yes no

Departure time

Arrival time

mask on others yes no

DATE:

your health:

NAMES
include people you traveled with

PLACE
& address

describe the social distancing

your health:

| | | | | | | | | | | | | | |
|---|---|---|---|---|---|---|---|---|---|---|---|---|---|
| **PLACE** & address | **NAMES** include people you traveled with | mask on others yes no | Arrival time | Departure time | washed hands before yes no | hand sanitizer before yes no | mask on you yes no | transportation | body temperature | outdoors or inside | # of people | washed hands after yes no | hand sanitizer after yes no |
| | describe the social distancing | | | | | | | | | | | | |



DATE:

your health:

| PLACE & address | NAMES include people you traveled with | mask on others yes no | Arrival time | Departure time | washed hands before yes no | hand sanitizer before yes no | mask on you yes no | transportation | body temperature | outdoors or inside | # of people | washed hands after yes no | hand sanitizer after yes no |
|---|---|---|---|---|---|---|---|---|---|---|---|---|---|
| | | | | | | | | | | | | | |

describe the social distancing



DATE:

hand sanitizer after yes no

washed hands after yes no

# of people

outdoors or inside

body temperature

transportation

mask on you yes no

hand sanitizer before yes no

washed hands before yes no

Departure time

Arrival time

mask on others yes no

DATE:

your health:

**PLACE**
& address

**NAMES**
include people you traveled with

describe the social distancing

your health:

| PLACE & address | NAMES include people you traveled with | mask on others yes no | Arrival time | Departure time | washed hands before yes no | hand sanitizer before yes no | mask on you yes no | transportation | body temperature | outdoors or inside | # of people | washed hands after yes no | hand sanitizer after yes no |
|---|---|---|---|---|---|---|---|---|---|---|---|---|---|
| | describe the social distancing | | | | | | | | | | | | |



DATE:

hand sanitizer after yes no

washed hands after yes no

# of people

outdoors or inside

body temperature

transportation

mask on you yes no

hand sanitizer before yes no

washed hands before yes no

Departure time

Arrival time

mask on others yes no

your health:

NAMES include people you traveled with

PLACE & address

describe the social distancing

DATE:

your health:

| PLACE & address | NAMES include people you traveled with | mask on others yes no | Arrival time | Departure time | washed hands before yes no | hand sanitizer before yes no | mask on you yes no | transportation | body temperature | outdoors or inside | # of people | washed hands after yes no | hand sanitizer after yes no |
|---|---|---|---|---|---|---|---|---|---|---|---|---|---|
| | | | | | | | | | | | | | |

describe the social distancing



DATE:

DATE:

your health:

| PLACE & address | NAMES include people you traveled with | mask on others yes no | Arrival time | Departure time | washed hands before yes no | hand sanitizer before yes no | mask on you yes no | transportation | body temperature | outdoors or inside | # of people | washed hands after yes no | hand sanitizer after yes no |
|---|---|---|---|---|---|---|---|---|---|---|---|---|---|
| | | | | | | | | | | | | | |

describe the social distancing

your health:

| PLACE & address | NAMES include people you traveled with | mask on others yes no | Arrival time | Departure time | washed hands before yes no | hand sanitizer before yes no | mask on you yes no | transportation | body temperature | outdoors or inside | # of people | washed hands after yes no | hand sanitizer after yes no |
|---|---|---|---|---|---|---|---|---|---|---|---|---|---|

describe the social distancing



DATE:

**your health:**

**PLACE**
& address

**NAMES**
include people you traveled with

describe the social distancing

mask on others yes no

**Arrival time**

**Departure time**

washed hands before yes no

hand sanitizer before yes no

mask on you yes no

transportation

body temperature

outdoors or inside

# of people

washed hands after yes no

hand sanitizer after yes no

**DATE:**

your health:

| PLACE & address | NAMES include people you traveled with | mask on others yes no | Arrival time | Departure time | washed hands before yes no | hand sanitizer before yes no | mask on you yes no | transportation | body temperature | outdoors or inside | # of people | washed hands after yes no | hand sanitizer after yes no |
|---|---|---|---|---|---|---|---|---|---|---|---|---|---|
| | | | | | | | | | | | | | |

describe the social distancing



DATE:

DATE:

hand sanitizer after yes no

washed hands after yes no

# of people

outdoors or inside

body temperature

transportation

mask on you yes no

hand sanitizer before yes no

washed hands before yes no

**Departure time**

**Arrival time**

mask on others yes no

**NAMES**
include people you traveled with

describe the social distancing

**PLACE**
& address

your health:

Contact Tracing LOG: A Logical Necessity™ 

your health:

| PLACE & address | NAMES include people you traveled with | mask on others yes no | Arrival time | Departure time | washed hands before yes no | hand sanitizer before yes no | mask on you yes no | transportation | body temperature | outdoors or inside | # of people | washed hands after yes no | hand sanitizer after yes no |
|---|---|---|---|---|---|---|---|---|---|---|---|---|---|
| | describe the social distancing | | | | | | | | | | | | |



DATE:

**DATE:**

hand sanitizer after yes no

washed hands after yes no

# of people

outdoors or inside

body temperature

transportation

mask on you yes no

hand sanitizer before yes no

washed hands before yes no

**Departure time**

**Arrival time**

mask on others yes no

**your health:**

**NAMES** include people you traveled with

**PLACE** & address

**describe the social distancing**

DATE:

PLACE & address

NAMES include people you traveled with

mask on others yes no

Arrival time

Departure time

washed hands before yes no

hand sanitizer before yes no

mask on you yes no

transportation

body temperature

outdoors or inside

# of people

washed hands after yes no

hand sanitizer after yes no

your health:

describe the social distancing

DATE:

your health:

**PLACE** & address

**NAMES** include people you traveled with

mask on others yes no

**Arrival time**

**Departure time**

washed hands before yes no

hand sanitizer before yes no

mask on you yes no

transportation

body temperature

outdoors or inside

# of people

washed hands after yes no

hand sanitizer after yes no

describe the social distancing

hand sanitizer after yes no

washed hands after yes no

# of people

outdoors or inside

body temperature

transportation

mask on you yes no

hand sanitizer before yes no

washed hands before yes no

**Departure time**

**Arrival time**

mask on others yes no

**DATE:**

**PLACE**
& address

**NAMES**
include people you traveled with

**your health:**

**describe the social distancing**

hand sanitizer after yes no

washed hands after yes no

# of people

outdoors or inside

body temperature

transportation

mask on you yes no

hand sanitizer before yes no

washed hands before yes no

**Departure time**

**Arrival time**

mask on others yes no

**DATE:**

your health:

**NAMES**
include people you traveled with

**PLACE**
& address

describe the social distancing

your health:

| **PLACE** & address | **NAMES** include people you traveled with | mask on others yes no | Arrival time | Departure time | washed hands before yes no | hand sanitizer before yes no | mask on you yes no | transportation | body temperature | outdoors or inside | # of people | washed hands after yes no | hand sanitizer after yes no |
|---|---|---|---|---|---|---|---|---|---|---|---|---|---|
| | | | | | | | | | | | | | |

describe the social distancing



**DATE:**

hand sanitizer after yes no

washed hands after yes no

# of people

outdoors or inside

body temperature

transportation

mask on you yes no

hand sanitizer before yes no

washed hands before yes no

**Departure time**

**Arrival time**

mask on others yes no

your health:

**NAMES**
include people you traveled with

describe the social distancing

**PLACE**
& address

**DATE:**

your health:

| PLACE & address | NAMES include people you traveled with | mask on others yes no | Arrival time | Departure time | washed hands before yes no | hand sanitizer before yes no | mask on you yes no | transportation | body temperature | outdoors or inside | # of people | washed hands after yes no | hand sanitizer after yes no |
|---|---|---|---|---|---|---|---|---|---|---|---|---|---|
| | describe the social distancing | | | | | | | | | | | | |



DATE:

hand sanitizer after yes no

washed hands after yes no

# of people

outdoors or inside

body temperature

transportation

mask on you yes no

hand sanitizer before yes no

washed hands before yes no

**Departure time**

**Arrival time**

mask on others yes no

DATE:

your health:

**NAMES**
include people you traveled with

**PLACE**
& address

describe the social distancing

your health:

| PLACE & address | NAMES include people you traveled with | mask on others yes no | Arrival time | Departure time | washed hands before yes no | hand sanitizer before yes no | mask on you yes no | transportation | body temperature | outdoors or inside | # of people | washed hands after yes no | hand sanitizer after yes no |
|---|---|---|---|---|---|---|---|---|---|---|---|---|---|
| | | | | | | | | | | | | | |

describe the social distancing



DATE:

hand sanitizer after yes no

washed hands after yes no

# of people

outdoors or inside

body temperature

transportation

mask on you yes no

hand sanitizer before yes no

washed hands before yes no

**Departure time**

**Arrival time**

mask on others yes no

your health:

**NAMES**
include people you traveled with

**PLACE**
& address

describe the social distancing

**DATE:**

your health:

| PLACE & address | NAMES include people you traveled with | mask on others yes no | Arrival time | Departure time | washed hands before yes no | hand sanitizer before yes no | mask on you yes no | transportation | body temperature | outdoors or inside | # of people | washed hands after yes no | hand sanitizer after yes no |
|---|---|---|---|---|---|---|---|---|---|---|---|---|---|
| | | | | | | | | | | | | | |

describe the social distancing



DATE:

hand sanitizer after yes no

washed hands after yes no

# of people

outdoors or inside

body temperature

transportation

mask on you yes no

hand sanitizer before yes no

washed hands before yes no

**Departure time**

**Arrival time**

mask on others yes no

**DATE:**

your health:

**NAMES** include people you traveled with

**PLACE** & address

describe the social distancing

your health:

| PLACE & address | NAMES include people you traveled with | mask on others yes no | Arrival time | Departure time | washed hands before yes no | hand sanitizer before yes no | mask on you yes no | transportation | body temperature | outdoors or inside | # of people | washed hands after yes no | hand sanitizer after yes no |
|---|---|---|---|---|---|---|---|---|---|---|---|---|---|
| | | | | | | | | | | | | | |

describe the social distancing



DATE:

your health:

PLACE
& address

NAMES
include people you traveled with

describe the social distancing

mask on others yes no

Arrival time

Departure time

washed hands before yes no

hand sanitizer before yes no

mask on you yes no

transportation

body temperature

outdoors or inside

# of people

washed hands after yes no

hand sanitizer after yes no

DATE:

your health:

| PLACE & address | NAMES include people you traveled with | mask on others yes no | Arrival time | Departure time | washed hands before yes no | hand sanitizer before yes no | mask on you yes no | transportation | body temperature | outdoors or inside | # of people | washed hands after yes no | hand sanitizer after yes no |
|---|---|---|---|---|---|---|---|---|---|---|---|---|---|
| | | | | | | | | | | | | | |

describe the social distancing



DATE:

DATE:

hand sanitizer after yes no

washed hands after yes no

# of people

outdoors or inside

body temperature

transportation

mask on you yes no

hand sanitizer before yes no

washed hands before yes no

Departure time

Arrival time

mask on others yes no

your health:

NAMES
include people you traveled with

PLACE
& address

describe the social distancing

hand sanitizer after yes no

washed hands after yes no

# of people

outdoors or inside

body temperature

transportation

mask on you yes no

hand sanitizer before yes no

washed hands before yes no

**Departure time**

**Arrival time**

mask on others yes no

**NAMES**
include people you traveled with

**PLACE**
& address

your health:

describe the social distancing

**DATE:**

hand sanitizer after yes no

washed hands after yes no

# of people

outdoors or inside

body temperature

transportation

mask on you yes no

hand sanitizer before yes no

washed hands before yes no

Departure time

Arrival time

mask on others yes no

DATE:

your health:

NAMES
include people you traveled with

PLACE
& address

describe the social distancing

your health:

| PLACE & address | NAMES include people you traveled with | mask on others yes no | Arrival time | Departure time | washed hands before yes no | hand sanitizer before yes no | mask on you yes no | transportation | body temperature | outdoors or inside | # of people | washed hands after yes no | hand sanitizer after yes no |
|---|---|---|---|---|---|---|---|---|---|---|---|---|---|
| | describe the social distancing | | | | | | | | | | | | |



DATE:

DATE:

your health:

PLACE
& address

NAMES
include people
you traveled with

describe the
social distancing

mask on others yes no

Arrival time

Departure time

washed hands before yes no

hand sanitizer before yes no

mask on you yes no

transportation

body temperature

outdoors or inside

# of people

washed hands after yes no

hand sanitizer after yes no

hand sanitizer after yes no

washed hands after yes no

# of people

outdoors or inside

body temperature

transportation

mask on you yes no

hand sanitizer before yes no

washed hands before yes no

Departure time

Arrival time

mask on others yes no

your health:

PLACE & address

NAMES include people you traveled with

describe the social distancing

DATE:

DATE:

your health:

**PLACE**
& address

**NAMES**
include people
you traveled with

describe the
social distancing

mask on others yes no

**Arrival time**

**Departure time**

washed hands before yes no

hand sanitizer before yes no

mask on you yes no

transportation

body temperature

outdoors or inside

# of people

washed hands after yes no

hand sanitizer after yes no

hand sanitizer after yes no

washed hands after yes no

# of people

outdoors or inside

body temperature

transportation

mask on you yes no

hand sanitizer before yes no

washed hands before yes no

Departure time

Arrival time

mask on others yes no

your health:

PLACE
& address

NAMES
include people
you traveled with

describe the
social distancing

DATE:

**DATE:**

**your health:**

| **PLACE** & address | **NAMES** include people you traveled with | mask on others yes no | Arrival time | Departure time | washed hands before yes no | hand sanitizer before yes no | mask on you yes no | transportation | body temperature | outdoors or inside | # of people | washed hands after yes no | hand sanitizer after yes no |
|---|---|---|---|---|---|---|---|---|---|---|---|---|---|
| | | | | | | | | | | | | | |

**describe the social distancing**

your health:

| PLACE & address | NAMES include people you traveled with | mask on others yes no | Arrival time | Departure time | washed hands before yes no | hand sanitizer before yes no | mask on you yes no | transportation | body temperature | outdoors or inside | # of people | washed hands after yes no | hand sanitizer after yes no |
|---|---|---|---|---|---|---|---|---|---|---|---|---|---|
| | | | | | | | | | | | | | |

describe the social distancing



DATE:

hand sanitizer after yes no

washed hands after yes no

# of people

outdoors or inside

body temperature

transportation

mask on you yes no

hand sanitizer before yes no

washed hands before yes no

Departure time

Arrival time

mask on others yes no

DATE:

your health:

**PLACE**
& address

**NAMES**
include people you traveled with

describe the social distancing

your health:

| PLACE & address | NAMES include people you traveled with | mask on others yes no | Arrival time | Departure time | washed hands before yes no | hand sanitizer before yes no | mask on you yes no | transportation | body temperature | outdoors or inside | # of people | washed hands after yes no | hand sanitizer after yes no |
|---|---|---|---|---|---|---|---|---|---|---|---|---|---|
| | | | | | | | | | | | | | |

describe the social distancing



DATE:

hand sanitizer after yes no

washed hands after yes no

# of people

outdoors or inside

body temperature

transportation

mask on you yes no

hand sanitizer before yes no

washed hands before yes no

Departure time

Arrival time

mask on others yes no

NAMES include people you traveled with

describe the social distancing

your health:

PLACE & address

DATE:

hand sanitizer after yes no

washed hands after yes no

# of people

outdoors or inside

body temperature

transportation

mask on you yes no

hand sanitizer before yes no

washed hands before yes no

**Departure time**

**Arrival time**

mask on others yes no

your health:

**NAMES** include people you traveled with

**PLACE** & address

describe the social distancing

**DATE:**

hand sanitizer after yes no

washed hands after yes no

# of people

outdoors or inside

body temperature

transportation

mask on you yes no

hand sanitizer before yes no

washed hands before yes no

**Departure time**

**Arrival time**

mask on others yes no

your health:

**NAMES**
include people you traveled with

**PLACE**
& address

describe the social distancing

**DATE:**

your health:

| PLACE & address | NAMES include people you traveled with | mask on others yes no | Arrival time | Departure time | washed hands before yes no | hand sanitizer before yes no | mask on you yes no | transportation | body temperature | outdoors or inside | # of people | washed hands after yes no | hand sanitizer after yes no |
|---|---|---|---|---|---|---|---|---|---|---|---|---|---|
| | | | | | | | | | | | | | |

describe the social distancing



DATE:

DATE:

hand sanitizer after yes no

washed hands after yes no

# of people

outdoors or inside

body temperature

transportation

mask on you yes no

hand sanitizer before yes no

washed hands before yes no

**Departure time**

**Arrival time**

mask on others yes no

**NAMES**
include people you traveled with

describe the social distancing

**PLACE**
& address

your health:

your health:

| PLACE & address | NAMES include people you traveled with | mask on others yes no | Arrival time | Departure time | washed hands before yes no | hand sanitizer before yes no | mask on you yes no | transportation | body temperature | outdoors or inside | # of people | washed hands after yes no | hand sanitizer after yes no |
|---|---|---|---|---|---|---|---|---|---|---|---|---|---|
| | | | | | | | | | | | | | |

describe the social distancing



DATE:

hand sanitizer after yes no

washed hands after yes no

# of people

outdoors or inside

body temperature

transportation

mask on you yes no

hand sanitizer before yes no

washed hands before yes no

Departure time

Arrival time

mask on others yes no

DATE:

your health:

NAMES include people you traveled with

PLACE & address

describe the social distancing

your health:

| PLACE & address | NAMES include people you traveled with | mask on others yes no | Arrival time | Departure time | washed hands before yes no | hand sanitizer before yes no | mask on you yes no | transportation | body temperature | outdoors or inside | # of people | washed hands after yes no | hand sanitizer after yes no |
|---|---|---|---|---|---|---|---|---|---|---|---|---|---|
| | | | | | | | | | | | | | |

describe the social distancing



DATE:

DATE:

your health:

**PLACE**
& address

**NAMES**
include people
you traveled with

describe the
social distancing

mask on others yes no

**Arrival time**

**Departure time**

washed hands before yes no

hand sanitizer before yes no

mask on you yes no

transportation

body temperature

outdoors or inside

# of people

washed hands after yes no

hand sanitizer after yes no

your health:

| PLACE & address | NAMES include people you traveled with | mask on others yes no | Arrival time | Departure time | washed hands before yes no | hand sanitizer before yes no | mask on you yes no | transportation | body temperature | outdoors or inside | # of people | washed hands after yes no | hand sanitizer after yes no |
|---|---|---|---|---|---|---|---|---|---|---|---|---|---|
| | | | | | | | | | | | | | |

describe the social distancing



DATE:

hand sanitizer after yes no

washed hands after yes no

# of people

outdoors or inside

body temperature

transportation

mask on you yes no

hand sanitizer before yes no

washed hands before yes no

Departure time

Arrival time

mask on others yes no

your health:

NAMES include people you traveled with

PLACE & address

describe the social distancing

DATE:

your health:

| PLACE & address | NAMES include people you traveled with | mask on others yes no | Arrival time | Departure time | washed hands before yes no | hand sanitizer before yes no | mask on you yes no | transportation | body temperature | outdoors or inside | # of people | washed hands after yes no | hand sanitizer after yes no |
|---|---|---|---|---|---|---|---|---|---|---|---|---|---|
| | | | | | | | | | | | | | |

describe the social distancing



DATE:

DATE:

hand sanitizer after yes no

washed hands after yes no

# of people

outdoors or inside

body temperature

transportation

mask on you yes no

hand sanitizer before yes no

washed hands before yes no

**Departure time**

**Arrival time**

mask on others yes no

**your health:**

**NAMES** include people you traveled with

**PLACE** & address

describe the social distancing

**DATE:**

**hand sanitizer after** yes no

**washed hands after** yes no

**# of people**

**outdoors or inside**

**body temperature**

**transportation**

**mask on you** yes no

**hand sanitizer before** yes no

**washed hands before** yes no

**Departure time**

**Arrival time**

**mask on others** yes no

**PLACE**
**& address**

**NAMES**
include people
you traveled with

**your health:**

**describe the**
**social distancing**

hand sanitizer after yes no

washed hands after yes no

# of people

outdoors or inside

body temperature

transportation

mask on you yes no

hand sanitizer before yes no

washed hands before yes no

Departure time

Arrival time

mask on others yes no

your health:

NAMES include people you traveled with

PLACE & address

describe the social distancing

DATE:

your health:

| PLACE & address | NAMES include people you traveled with | mask on others yes no | Arrival time | Departure time | washed hands before yes no | hand sanitizer before yes no | mask on you yes no | transportation | body temperature | outdoors or inside | # of people | washed hands after yes no | hand sanitizer after yes no |
|---|---|---|---|---|---|---|---|---|---|---|---|---|---|
| | | | | | | | | | | | | | |

describe the social distancing



DATE:

hand sanitizer after yes no

washed hands after yes no

# of people

outdoors or inside

body temperature

transportation

mask on you yes no

hand sanitizer before yes no

washed hands before yes no

Departure time

Arrival time

mask on others yes no

DATE:

PLACE & address

NAMES include people you traveled with

describe the social distancing

your health:

hand sanitizer after yes no

washed hands after yes no

# of people

outdoors or inside

body temperature

transportation

mask on you yes no

hand sanitizer before yes no

washed hands before yes no

Departure time

Arrival time

mask on others yes no

NAMES include people you traveled with

PLACE & address

your health:

describe the social distancing

DATE:

hand sanitizer after yes no

washed hands after yes no

# of people

outdoors or inside

body temperature

transportation

mask on you yes no

hand sanitizer before yes no

washed hands before yes no

Departure time

Arrival time

mask on others yes no

your health:

NAMES

include people you traveled with

PLACE

& address

describe the social distancing

DATE:

hand sanitizer after yes no

washed hands after yes no

# of people

outdoors or inside

body temperature

transportation

mask on you yes no

hand sanitizer before yes no

washed hands before yes no

**Departure time**

**Arrival time**

mask on others yes no

**DATE:**

your health:

**PLACE**
& address

**NAMES**
include people you traveled with

describe the social distancing

hand sanitizer after yes no

washed hands after yes no

# of people

outdoors or inside

body temperature

transportation

mask on you yes no

hand sanitizer before yes no

washed hands before yes no

DATE:

**Departure time**

**Arrival time**

mask on others yes no

your health:

**NAMES**
include people you traveled with

describe the social distancing

**PLACE**
& address

your health:

| PLACE & address | NAMES include people you traveled with | mask on others yes no | Arrival time | Departure time | washed hands before yes no | hand sanitizer before yes no | mask on you yes no | transportation | body temperature | outdoors or inside | # of people | washed hands after yes no | hand sanitizer after yes no |
|---|---|---|---|---|---|---|---|---|---|---|---|---|---|
| | | | | | | | | | | | | | |

describe the
social distancing



DATE:

DATE:

hand sanitizer after yes no

washed hands after yes no

# of people

outdoors or inside

body temperature

transportation

mask on you yes no

hand sanitizer before yes no

washed hands before yes no

**Departure time**

**Arrival time**

mask on others yes no

your health:

**NAMES**
include people you traveled with

**PLACE**
& address

describe the social distancing

Made in United States
North Haven, CT
05 November 2026

21768937R00135